HOW TO CURE

BAD BREATH

How To Cure Bad Breath

Understanding The Causes Of Bad Breath
And The Cure For Bad Breath

Alan Le Blanc

TABLE OF CONTENT

The Bad Breath Problem

Bad breath happens when there is a smelly and distasteful odour which comes out from the mouth. This happens when someone exhales. When they exhale, the odour would come out, thus causing the bad breath problem.

This is not only a health issue, but a social issue as well. Many people are turned off by people who have bad breath because the moment they open their mouth, the odour can be smelt. It is something which the sufferer denies but those around them would be able to smell their breath.

In this book, you would learn about the various causes of bad breath as well as the best treatments for them. Bad breath is an issue which you can't deal just on the surface. You would need to deal with it internally as well.

In the chapter, you would learn about how you can check if you have bad breath and the potential causes of your bad breath.

Checking For Bad Breath

Many people deny that they have bad breath. Their loved ones may have told them about this problem but they have problem in accepting that their breath stinks.

Anyone who has a loved one with this problem would know how difficult it is to tell another person. In the later chapters, I would teach you how you can tell them that they have bad breath without getting a bad reaction from them.

Therefore, if you suspect that you have bad breath, there are several ways of determining if you have bad breath.

Among the ways include:

- **Breathe On The Back Of Your Hands**. This is the easiest method of determining if you have bad breathe. Simply smell the odour as it comes out from your mouth. This could determine quickly if your breath smells terrible.

- **Use A Spoon Or Tongue Scraper**. Use either of them to test your breath. Simply scrape your tongue at the back and front of your tongue. Do each area one at a time and smell the area on the spoon or scraper. See how it smells. If it smells bad, then you may have a chronic bad breath (halitosis) problem.

- **Check Your Saliva**. Are you aware that saliva has odour? If you don't know, you do now. Your hope is that when you conduct this test, your breath would stop having a foul odour. To perform this, just slightly lick your wrist or the back of your hand.

  Give a few seconds and then smelling it. If you don't smell anything, it is alright. If it does smell, check with your dentist and get the help that you need.

- **Black Spots On Your Teeth**. Simply check if you have any black spots on your teeth. If you do, it is a sign that you have bad breath. This may also be a sign that you have gum and tooth problems that would lead to bad breath due to the formed bacteria.

You would need to consult a dentist to provide the proper treatment for those areas that affected you so you can cure your bad breath problem.

Halitosis is a major problem when you have chronic bad breath. It is worse when it is chronic. Regardless of whether it happens a few times or a problem which never seems to end, people would find for a way to get rid of it.

There are various reasons for bad breath. Among them include:

- **Dental Issues** - Poor dental hygiene causes periodontal disease which can also cause bad breath. If you don't brush and floss daily, the food particle would remain in your mouth.

You would probably need to brush and floss a few times a day in order to ensure that your mouth is clean. If food particles remain in your mouth, they would absorb bacteria.

From here, you may experience plague in your teeth. If you don't brush your teeth properly, this plague affects your gums. You may end up getting either gingivitis or tooth decay.

Pockets could form between your teeth and gums. This is known as the periodontitis condition which can cause bad breath to linger.

- **Food** - While eating, the food particles which remain in and around your teeth could cause an odour in your mouth. Everyone would know that onions and garlic are perhaps the worst culprits of this condition.

  Once these foods and smelly oils are digested, they would penetrate into your blood. From there, it would travel to your lungs and come up to your breath when you open your mouth. The smell could linger up to five days.

- **Dry Mouth Problem** - Generally, the inside of your mouth should be moist with saliva. Saliva plays a role of cleaning your mouth. When you don't have any saliva circulating inside your mouth, the dead cells would gather on your tongue.

They could also come on your cheeks and gums. This is known as having dry mouth. As soon as the dead cells accumulate, they would deteriorate and cause a foul smell inside the mouth.

This condition would happen when the person is sleeping. If you sleep with your mouth open, you are more prone to having a dry mouth. The moment you wake up in the morning, it could also cause 'morning breath' problems.

- **Nose And Throat Infections** - Bad breath can also happen when the person has certain allergies. Sinus infections would cause a nasal discharge. It would go from the back of your throat and slowly trickles downwards.

This causes a foul odour. You could also have bad breath if you have certain upper respiratory ailments which make you cough up mucus.

- **Chronic Diseases** - You can also emit foul odours when you have certain chronic lung ailments like infections and abscesses. It would emit foul odours when you open your mouth.

Besides that, if you have a chronic kidney failure, you can also have a certain mouth odour which smells like urine. When you have a fishy odour, it could mean that you have a chronic liver ailment.

Meanwhile, those who have diabetes have a fruity odour. Besides that, those who have stomach ailment are also often linked to having bad breathe.

- **Smoking Tobacco** - Those who smoke cigarettes are also prone to bad breath. This happens because when you smoke cigarettes, your mouth would be dry. Besides that, smoking would also cause an unpleasant odour after puffing a cigarette. If you are someone who smokes, there is a greater possibility that you get periodontal disease - a cause for bad breath.

- **Milk** - Some people can't tolerate milk. If you find out that you are one of those people, tend you need to get rid of it. You would develop bad breath if you are consuming milk or dairy products that you can't digest.

- **Extreme Dieting** - If you are on a special diet or fasting in order to lose weight, you would also have bad breath. This happens as you develop ketoacidosis, which is a situation where the chemicals break down while you are fasting.

- **Alcohol** - Drinking alcohol not only causes multiple health issues, but would also heavily impact your digestive system. When your digestive system is problematic, it causes dry mouth and this leads to further bad breath problems.

- **Stress** - It may be hard for you to believe it, but stress is a big factor in bad breath. If you are stressed out, your digestion would be affected and this triggers further bad breath.

Nonetheless, those with normal fresh breath also could develop halitosis over time. Among the other various causes of bad breath include:

- Usage of drugs
- Cavities
- Dentures
- Insulin
- Gingivitis
- Tonsils which catch food particles
- Vitamin supplements
- Cancer of the mouth or throat
- Dehydration
- HIV infection

If you find yourself having any of these situations, you could look to cure those situations. Find for the proper solutions to ensure that you have a better quality of breath.

How To Get Rid Of Bad Breath

In this chapter are some methods of alleviating bad breath. Some are simple while some are more complicated and may even require some extra costs associated with.

However, many of those costs that you have to spend is nothing compared to the benefits of having alleviating your bad breath.

In the next few chapters, I would share all about alleviating bad breath. Some are permanent while some are only temporary.

Oral Hygiene

It is important that you maintain a regular oral hygiene. This isn't just important for your dental health but for your regular health as well.

With proper oral hygiene, there are three areas of your mouth which you should focus on: the gums, tongue and teeth. The most common oral hygiene is to simply brush and floss your teeth twice each day, one in the morning and one at night.

These are the oral hygiene habits that you should have:

- **Floss at least once a day**. If possible, floss even more. Flossing is an important part of oral hygiene because it helps remove food particles which are stuck in your teeth.

Besides that, it also would help if you remove the plaque. It is extremely important to get rid of plaque on your teeth because it could not only cause periodontal disease, but also heart disease and other heart ailments.

- **Brush your teeth after you eat**. If you work away from home, always make it a point to brush after you eat at the workplace. Your colleagues may find it weird, but tell them that you are practicing good oral hygiene.

- **Brush every part of your mouth**. It may sound weird, but brushing your teeth can remove the dead cells from your tongue. Besides that, it is also very helpful in removing leftover food particles and bacteria.

To perform this, simply use a toothbrush with softer bristle or a tongue scraper. Try to go as far back into the mouth as you can without gagging. You will be amazed that most of the bacteria are towards the back.

- **Toothbrush with small bristles**. When you brush, use those with small bristles. You need to also change your toothbrush every four months to ensure that it still effective in cleaning out the leftover food.

- **Clean your dentures**. If you wear dentures, you need to make sure that they are cleaned thoroughly. Ideally, they should be cleaned at least once a day.

- **Regular Dentist Check-Up**. Make sure that you see a dentist on a regular basis. The general advice is to have your teeth checked and cleaned twice a year.

- **Fill Your Cavities**. If you have cavities in your teeth, quickly make an appointment with your dentist to have them filled. Cavities are an opening to allow bacteria in. This in turn, causes bad breath.

- **Use A Waterpik**. After breakfast, it is very helpful to clean your mouth and wash away any food particles which are left behind.

- **Swish Water In Your Mouth**. After eating a meal, you should swish water in your mouth. You wouldn't be able to get rid of certain food particles that were stuck in your teeth regardless of how hard you try. As such water helps to clean certain parts that normal brushing or flossing isn't able to reach.

- **Use Natural Oral Hygiene Remedies**. With the use of natural oral hygiene remedies, you would be able to get rid of bad breath as well. Preferably, try to use baking soda and hydrogen peroxide as they can work wonders.
Using antiseptic tree oil or eucalyptus oil can be also very helpful to sanitize your mouth. Simply add a little oil on your toothbrush. If you feel that is too much a hassle, you can simply head to a health

food store to purchase natural toothpaste remedies.

- **Sanitize Your Toothbrush**. This can be done by placing your toothbrush in a container of hydrogen peroxide to ensure that your toothbrush is bacteria-free. The moment you are ready to brush your teeth, you would need to rinse your toothbrush well.

- **Use Fresh Parsley Or Small Mint**. Simply put a small portion of either sugarless small mint or fresh parsley in your mouth. This easily helps you improve the smell your breath.

- **Free Your Mouth From Food Particles**. Try to ensure that food doesn't stick in your teeth or pocket areas.

- **Don't Eat Spicy Food With Onions And Garlic**.

- **Drink Lots Of Water**. By drinking a lot of water, you would be able to keep your mouth moist. Besides that, you could also produce saliva by chewing sugarless gum or candy. If your mouth is constantly dry, you should get a prescription of artificial saliva preparation or oral medications which produces saliva in your mouth.

- **Use Tongue Scrapers**. There are people who use tongue scrapers to remove bad breath. They could be purchased from pharmacies and come in different size.

  This is placed at the back of your tongue and then gently scraps it. This is repeated as many times as needed. Many people have used this method effectively in removing bad breathe.

However, this could be done by using a toothbrush as well. Regardless, it is more important to have dental hygiene which is regular. Ensure that you brush your tongue after you eat.

- **Keep The Bacteria Away By Drinking More Water**. This helps to keep the bacteria away as it ensures that saliva is in your mouth.

- **Don't Use Mouthwash**. This may be a shocking tip but it's true. Try not to get mouthwash from drugstores as they normally contain alcohol. It dries your mouth and produces bacteria at the same time.

Besides that, mouthwash that has more than 25% of alcohol could contribute to oral cancer. Try finding for mouthwash which has a mixture of at least half hydrogen peroxide and half water. Take it and gargle for about 30 seconds for best effect.

- **Use Mouthwash**. This may contradict the previous point, but mouthwash is highly effective in cleaning bacteria which is underneath your tongue.

  Besides that, you could also find bacteria on your throat and tonsils. It is hard to get rid of them. As such, you should still use mouthwash, only one which doesn't contain alcohol.

- **Stop Smoking**. If you are someone who smokes, stop this habit. Products related to tobacco aren't good for your health, and better breath.

- **Gargle Constantly**. Start gargling as soon as you can. You can simply use water. Gargling is great because there are certain difficult places where the bacteria could creep in while sleeping. Gargle for a minimum of 30 seconds every morning and try to get as close as possible to the bottom of your throat. Ensure that your rinse your mouth well to ensure that your remove all the bacteria and other elements. You should also do this after every meal, if possible.

- **Mix Water With Salt**. Salt is incredible in killing with bacteria. By simply mixing salt with water, and gargling with it, this would help your eliminate bad breath and halitosis.

Watch Out On The Food You Eat

Certain foods are more susceptible to bad breath than others. This includes foods which are high in fat, loaded with sugar, meats, specialty and certain dairy products. It is important to note that foods which contain acid would produce more bacteria in your mouth.

When eating foods with a lot of fats or protein, they may find it difficult to digest them properly. Those who have problem digesting meat and dairy products would end up having bad breath. These are certain suggestions on food to improve your bad breath.

- **Avoid Coffee And Certain Tea**. Coffee and certain teas are culprits of bad breath problem. Both have plenty of acid and try to stop drinking so much of it.

  However, drinking black tea helps keep bacteria way and is helpful in improving your breath. Besides that, you could also help prevent bad breath with green tea or peppermint tea.

  Tea could also remove the bad breath caused by mucus. You simply need to drink a cup a day to ensure that the odour would slowly dissipate.

- **Eat Fruits And Vegetables**. They are rich for antioxidants. This would include eating broccoli, cabbage, berries and leafy greens. They not only ensure your health but also ensure that your bad breath doesn't occur.

- **Eat Sugar-Free Yogurt**. Yogurt which is sugar-free and has a live culture helps keep away the bacteria responsible for bad breath.

- **Remove Certain Spices From Your Diet**. Besides onion and garlic, spices like curry could cause people to have bad breath. When digesting them, certain elements would flow through the bloodstream and to the lungs. This odour would be emitted in about 24 hours.

Taking Supplements Or Vitamins

- **Lack Of Vitamin B**. This is a major cause of bad breath. Find for proper supplements to take which has Vitamin B.

- **A Lack Of Zinc**. If you have zinc deficiency, you need to take more than 60mg in a day. However, don't take too much as zinc could interfere with copper.

- **Lack Of Vitamin C**. If you take in lesser than 6000mg of Vitamin B, you would remove the mucus and toxins which are built up in your body. They are stored up in your body and are a major cause of bad breath.

Improve Your Digestion

Another major cause of bad breath is your digestive system. You would most definitely need to improve it by watching what you eat.

You have to be very careful about the food you eat because eating the wrong food wouldn't help eliminate bad breath. Among the tips to ensure that your digestive system is intact includes:

- **High-Fibre Diet**. Having a diet filled with high fibre including whole grains, vegetables and fresh food would ensure that you digest better than having a diet which isn't high with fibre.

- **Take Enzyme Tablets**. If you don't have sufficient enzymes to ensure proper digestion, you would need to take more than four enzyme tablets after each major meal.

- **Lack Of Hydrochloric Acid**. To ensure that you have more hydrochloric acid, you could try using apple cider vinegar. Try taking one tablespoon before a major meal. Use betaine or pepsin tablets before you eat to ensure your digestion works better.

- **Drink More Water**. Drinking at least eight glasses of water each day ensures that you eliminate bad breath from a lack of regular bowel movement.

The Power Of Herbal Remedies

- Use Alfalfa Tablets
- Basil, rosemary, parsley and thyme
- Place fennel on your gums and tongues to remove bad breath
- Make tea with cloves. Simply use three whole cloves or ground, combine with hot water and allow it to sit for around 20 minutes.
- Lemon wedge with salt would help you if taking onions or garlic.
- Chew natural gums which have spearmint or peppermint oils. They could eliminate bacterium which causes bad breath. When chewing the gum, it

produces saliva which helps get rid of the bad breath.

- Gargle with a teaspoon of honey and cinnamon powder. Combine with hot water. This is a remedy that should be done in the morning to keep your breath fresh for the whole day.

- Use peppermint to calm your stomach. Simply place the peppermint into the tea in order to calm your stomach. You simply exhale through the lungs and from there; your breath would have a nice sweet smell to it.

- Chew sage. This helps you remove your bad breath as sage has oils with an antibacterial element that assists in removing the foul odour.

- Tea Tree Oil. It comes from the Melaleuca plant and its oil has certain elements which could disinfect your mouth and remove the bacteria. This can be found in certain toothpaste.

For some people, using herbs would work better because their system isn't abrasive to it. They aren't only natural, but it taken orally, it would affect your blood and provide a relief for your bad breath.

Certain other relief may help eliminate bad breath, but they create certain side effects to your body and pores. Herbal remedies work not only for your breath, but help make your health better.

However, it should be noted that herbal remedies won't cover up the bad breath issue. They simply work to remove the cause of it. It helps pinpoint what triggers your breath to smell bad. To ensure that herbal remedies work at its best, you should treat the cause of the problem to remove it.

By using herbal remedies, you can also change the way you eat and what you eat. If you are someone who consumes a lot of red meat or dairy products, there is a higher possibility of you having bad breath.

Using Chinese herbs

Chinese medication has a long ancient history. Many people have used them successfully in curing certain ailments they are afflicted with. A great majority of those treatments use Chinese herbs and tackling bad breath is one of those ailments that can be cured.

Among the types of herb used to remove bad breath include honeysuckle, gypsum and bamboo leaves. As there are so many Chinese herbs, you should first consult your physician first. You may even ask someone who has experience with Chinese herbs to provide a proper solution.

Using Breath Spray

There are some people who choose to use breath spray to remove bad breath. This may work or not. If you have chronic bad breath problems, it can be because of some sort of deeper because which breath spray simply won't help. Breath spray is just a temporary fix. If it is caused by something internal, using breath spray wouldn't help at all. It just masks the problem.

If you have digestion problems with bad breath, the advice is to see a physician to see what the real problem is. It can be that there is a more serious issue than simply bad breath.

You should only use breath spray if your bad breath is temporary. When finding for a type of breath spray to use, find for one which doesn't contain alcohol. Alcohol is something which can work for and against you. It may get rid of bad breath bacteria, but it also makes your mouth dry.

It may take some time to find a breath spray that suits you. However, it is very important that you find a breath spray which is oil-based rather than alcohol-based. Based on my experience, the best kind of breath spray would be one which contains peppermint or eucalyptus oil.

You should be clear that this only works temporarily. You can't just depend on breath spray but also practice good oral hygiene every day. This includes flossing and brushing your teeth well. This helps maintain your oral health and prevent bad breath from recurring.

Should You Use Over-The-Counter (OTC) Medications

Most people who want a quick fix for their bad breath issue would head directly to a drugstore to get over the counter medication. This is the normal thing that most people do. However, if you don't really know much about the product you are using, you are simply wasting your time and money.

There are plenty of medications in the drugstore which are used for bad breath and you wouldn't need a prescription to get them. However, they are not guarantees in eliminating bad breath from your system.

The reason for bad breath differs between individuals and you may not even know the reason for your bad breath in the first place. There are multiple types of bad breath and you would need a different kind of treatment for each. If you don't know the deeper cause of it, you wouldn't be able to get rid of your bad breath like you want.

For this, you should consult a physician to ensure that you know the deeper cause of your bad breath. You might need to get something stronger and more effective than the most common over-the-counter medication.

Most of the time over-the-counter medication isn't as powerful as medication prescribed by your physician. This is because over-the-counter medications normally use natural products, which are normally slower in healing the condition.

They won't contain certain ingredients like antibiotics. You normally get antibiotics through prescription. However, you should remember that over-the-counter medication normally only provide limited and temporary relief.

Using Flaxseed For Bad Breath

Flaxseed is incredibly powerful for people with bad breath. However, this depends on the cause of your bad breath, first of all. We would look first at how flaxseed is produced.

Flaxseed is helpful in removing bad breath because of its Omega-3 properties that it has. Using Omega-3 fatty acids could be easily used to help remove your bad breath. It has important oils which provide nutrients to your body.

It would use oils and supplements that the body uses to remove bad breath. If you suffer from chronic halitosis, you could also use flaxseed because it has plenty of fatty acid which can fight bacteria which causes bad breath.

The Quickest Remedies For Bad Breath

Are you someone who goes to social events and you feel like your breath doesn't smell right? Or you might be in a meeting and supposed to meet a big client or your boss?

In such social situations, you may be self-conscious about the smell of your breath. It is of course impossible to not talk. As such, you would need to think of fast remedies which would help you get rid of your bad breath.

These are among some ways you can look to remove your bad breath:

- **Drink Water**. I may have mentioned this tip in the previous chapters and that is because it is incredibly important. Water has tremendous power in cleaning your mouth over a period of time. You would have fresher breath, especially if you need to talk to someone soon.

  If you have a dry mouth, it also helps to drink water to ensure that your mouth is moist. Dry mouth and bad breath normally comes together because of the bacteria which are formed inside. You can squeeze some lemon or lime to give it some flavour.

- **Rinse Your Mouth**. Rinsing your mouth should be done regularly if you have bad breath.

- **Chew Candy or Gum**. This would help you at the very last minute. If you can find one, quickly put it in your mouth. This ensures that your breath is fresh for a certain amount of time. However, ensure that you throw the gum once you are done. It is very irritating to talk to someone chewing a gum.

- **Eat Parsley**. If you don't have any mint or gum while you are out eating, parsley is another alternative. Parsley is normally used for decorating your meal. However, don't do this in front of anyone. Excuse yourself and head to the bathroom. Chew on the parsley for a few minutes and make sure that you rinse your mouth before going back. You wouldn't want other people to see green particles on your teeth as it is gross.

- **Brush Your Teeth**. If you have access to a toothbrush, you can brush your teeth immediately. This is great if you are near your destination and near a restroom.

- **Scrape Your Tongue**. A tongue scraper is also a quick alternative. However, you should always do this in private. Try finding a bathroom before attempting to do this. If you have any white spots on your tongue, remove them with a scraper or spoon.

- **A Small Shot Of Whisky Helps**. Yes, you heard it right. Drinking a small shot of whisky helps get rid of your bad breath for a moment.

It is believed that whiskey could get rid of certain germs that are on your teeth. This doesn't mean that you should drink alcohol mindlessly, especially at work. This is just to share the knowledge that whisky does improve your bad breath, if taken moderately.

Should You Seek Medical Assistance

If you can seem to have bad breath for a long period and just can seem to figure out why, then consulting a physician might be the way. This bad breath problem may be more than just your breath; it may have to do with a health ailment that you aren't even aware of.

Tell your physician about your problem and what you have tried to do to deal with it. He would ask you certain question pertaining to your health.

Among the main questions would be:

- Are you experiencing other health issues?
- Do you smoke?
- Do you take spicy food regularly?
- What is the smell of your breath or odour?
- Have you been practicing healthy oral hygiene?
- Have you tried any bad breath remedies?
- Do you have any problems with your dental hygiene?
- Do you have any allergies, sore throat or sinus problems?
- Do you have any other health issues?

After asking you these questions, the physician would examine you. He would check your nose and mouth. If you have a sore throat or mouth sores, they might need to get a culture. At times, additional tests are needed. You may need to have a chest x-ray, abdomen x-ray, endoscopy and thorough blood test.

If it is decided that you would need to see a dentist, the dentist would have to perform a thorough inspection of your mouth. To do that, the dentist may use a certain instrument to test for bad breath. A popular instrument is called the halimeter.

Halimeter is a machine which is used to record readings of your breath using a tube. You simply blow into the tube, similar to a breathalyzer machine. If it is suspected that you have bad breath or chronic halitosis, the dentist may test your breath regularly.

Besides that, the dentist would also determine what the cause of your bad breath is. Among the common causes would be having dimethyl sulphide and hydrogen sulphide. As you know the chemicals which cause your bad breath condition, you could make the changes to what you do daily.

The dentist would also see the chemicals and enzymes that are in your breath and they would be able to provide a proper treatment for your condition. However, this procedure could only be done in a dentist's office.

Together with the halimeter, your dentist may decide to use other testing as well. This includes gas chromatography and BANA tests.

Smokers And Bad Breath

If you are someone who live with or always with people who smoke, the smell may not bother you. You would not want to be in close proximity of someone who smokes because of their breath, if you are someone who isn't used to the smell. The smoker's breath could easily irritate you because it is incredibly strong.

Smokers who have bad breath can have the smell linger over a long period or could be very constant, especially for those who are chain smokers. Certain people wish they could stay way but they wouldn't want to hurt the smoker's feelings.

There are certain things however, that smokers could do to relieve themselves and others of the strong cigarette smell. This includes:

- **Chew Gum**. A smoker can hide their bad breath from smoking is to simply chew gum. Try getting a flavour which is strong and which would last for a moment. Or not, you can simply chew gums which are sugar-free.

  Besides that, sugar-free gum is better for your teeth. As teeth and related areas could affect your breath, chewing gum is perhaps the best way to go. You could also try getting specialty gum which is specially made for smokers, although they are a bit more expensive.

- **Get Mints**. Try getting mints which have long lasting flavour. They could last long enough for the smell to go away.

- **Use Mouthwash**. Smokers need to use mouthwash regularly to ensure that they are able to smell better than previously.

- Stop Smoking Altogether. If you really want to stop the nicotine breath, you should simply kick the habit.

From there, you can work on ensuring that your breath is fresh and getting rid of your bad breath.

You would also be healthier over a period of time.

Prevent Or Stop Bad Breath

In the earlier parts of this book, I have noted that chronic halitosis is caused when you don't have a regular or proper oral hygiene. Ideally, you should look to brush and floss your teeth twice a day - in the morning and before you sleep. This is the normal oral hygiene practice that everyone should follow.

However, if you are someone with bad breath, you can work to ensure that you start this oral practice as soon as you can. This is an important step towards curing bad breath once and for all.

How To Floss

Flossing helps to clean your teeth in certain areas where your toothbrush can't get to. These areas include the pockets and anywhere else where it is hard your toothbrush to reach. The pockets are simply the space between your teeth.

Unknown to most people, it is better to floss first and then only use your toothbrush. Most people brush first and then only floss later. If you do brush first, you may miss certain spots between your teeth. Once you have food sitting there, it would turn into plaque.

If the plaque isn't removed on time, it would cause your teeth to rod. You may end up with gum or periodontal disease.

What flossing does is to remove the food particles which are stuck between your teeth while you eat. Besides that, flossing could also help you in your cardiovascular health and dental health.

If you are someone who flosses regularly, you also help prevent the probability of heart attack and stroke. These are all very good reasons why you should have a daily dental hygiene routine.

To floss effectively, you simply place the floss in those spaces between your teeth. Move the floss within the space in an up and down motion. In order to remove all the particles, you should floss all the sides your teeth.

If you aren't sure about what to use, your dentist would be able to help you decide on the right flossing tools to use on your teeth. There are various kinds of floss available in the market. There are waxes or unwaxed floss. There are also different strengths from super thin to super strong.

Besides that, there is also flavoured floss. From peppermint to regular mint, all of them are tasty. However, don't just floss for the taste! You could also get dental floss holders if you want something proper to hold the floss in.

As you go to a dentist for a check-up, you may even get complimentary floss from them. Ideally, waxed floss is better because they are easier to use and your breath would smell minty fresh after use.

How To Brush

Many people fail to understand how to brush their teeth properly. You couldn't just go over them once and think that you are done with it. Many people don't take enough time to brush their teeth thoroughly. As such, it leaves particles in their teeth which are difficult to get out, even by regular flossing.

It is very common for people to be too busy that they don't have any time to brush their teeth well. If you brush too quickly, it would lead to plaque and bacteria setting in. It could lead to other dental problems in the future.

The best way to brush your teeth is to have your toothbrush at a 45 degree angle. This is a step by step approach towards brushing your teeth well:

- **Brush from bottom up**. Simply start from your lower gums and go upwards until you reach the top of your lower teeth.

- **Brush downwards**. Start from the top of your lower teeth to your lower gums. Brush your teeth on the outside using this same method. Brushing in a similar manner helps to remove the plaque from your gums.

If plaque hits your gums, it would cause gum disease. Besides that, you should also brush where you chew in a horizontal direction. And then, brush the chewing surfaces of your teeth in a horizontal movement.

To see quality results, you should ensure that you do floss and brush regularly. If not, the chances of you getting rid of bad breath are slim.

Why You Should Always Brush Your Tongue

As stated in previous chapters, brushing your tongue helps get rid of bad breath over time. To see the best results, you should do this properly. This could be easily done by using a toothbrush, although you can easily buy other instruments which could help you brush your tongue. It should never be something abrasive which can make you lose your taste buds.

The proper method of brushing your tongue is to simply take your toothbrush or instrument and gently place it at the back of your tongue. Try getting it as far back as possible. If you are doing it for the first time, you may cough or gag a little. However, this is the main area that you would want to focus on as there are a lot of bacteria and germs located at the back of your tongue. When brushing, you should also include the sides of your tongue.

Once you are done brushing your tongue, rinse your mouth a couple of time. Make sure that you do this properly as you need to remove any residue which remains in your mouth. This would include any food particles which you don't get in the first time around.

If you are going to brush your tongue, make sure to do it each time you brush your teeth. If you find it too time consuming to do that, try doing it for at least one time a day. You don't have to scrub your tongue with force. Simply a few brushes with your toothbrush or tongue scraper could do wonders, if done consistently.

Regardless, you should never forget about using your regular oral hygiene. Make sure to floss every single day. Stay away from acidic food as well as they tend to eliminate the enamel on your teeth.

When rinsing your mouth, use a mouthwash which doesn't have alcohol. Tongue brushing would be for nothing if you don't have a good oral habit. If practiced consistently, you would start to see immediate results, once implemented regularly.

Helping Others Who Have Bad Breath

Helping other with bad breath is perhaps one of the hardest things to do in life. Most of us are brought up to be nice to others, and telling someone that their breath stinks isn't easy.

In this chapter, we would look methods to tell someone that they have bad breath. Remember that this is something that is very contentious.

Helping Children With Bad Breath

Bad breath isn't limited to adults but children as well. There are certain children who have to deal with the problem of chronic halitosis as well. However, there isn't as many causes to bad breath like other adults would have.

Regardless, parents would still need to find out the chief reason behind their children's bad breath. This is important because if other children find out, they may end up teasing or distancing themselves from the child affected with bad breath.

Most of the time, bad breath in children is caused because of a lack of proper dental hygiene. If not monitored while they are brushing their teeth, they end up either not brushing properly, or may not even brush at all.

By not brushing, they may leave certain food particles in their mouth and if it stays there, turns into bacteria. When mixed with the saliva in the mouth, it would cause this bad breath problem.

Make sure that your children brush their teeth on a regular basis. If not, they would end up having bad breath throughout the day. Similar to adults, children should brush their teeth every morning and before their bedtime.

Children can also have cavities and if they are superficial, is another cause of bad breath in children. Besides that, they may also develop certain allergies like sinusitis or throat infection.

Sinus problems can arise when mucus clogs into the pharynx. They may develop a dry cough which keeps them up at the middle of the night. Their eyes would also itch and they may even have a running nose.

It is important that parents teach their children proper oral hygiene from a tender age. They need to advice their child on why is it important to brush their teeth as well as the proper method of doing it. Make sure that they understand the importance of having clean teeth throughout the day.

For young children, it is not recommended for them to use mouthwash. It may not be effective in ensuring their teeth are clean and may also be dangerous to them. This is because regular mouthwash has alcohol. If swallowed, would cause health risks for them and may even bring about death.

Check with your children if they know the right method of brushing. If not teach them the right way. You should also take them for regular dental check-up. Ideally, you should ensure that they check their teeth every half a year. If you start taking them to a dentist from a young age, they would learn to take care of their teeth better over time.

Dating Someone With Bad Breath

How would you feel if when you start talking to your date and find out that he/she has this bad breath problem?

This is perhaps something which is very hard to do - Dating someone with bad breath.

You would be shocked, wouldn't you. If you are someone nice, you would definitely resist against saying anything. However, this would perhaps be the last date that you have with them.

What if that person is you instead? Instead of your date having the bad breath, you are the one having it.

It is crucial that your breath is free of any foul odours. If suffering from chronic halitosis, you would need to correct the problem immediately before going on your date. If I am you, I wouldn't even want to be talking to anyone for at least a period of time.

If you have gone well with the date and about to land a kiss, you should make sure that your breath is fresh. If you don't have a fresh breath, you can easily turn off your date. They might not want to ever go out with you again or you may not want to go out with them ever again.

You should always work to ensure that you have a fresh breath, especially if you know you have this problem. If you are someone who doesn't have a proper oral hygiene, it is very important for you to develop one immediately. If you don't, going out on dates would be a very difficult thing.

If you are someone who smokes regularly and looking to date, make sure that you have gums or mints with you at all time. The smoker's breath is one of the worst smells I know of.

It is not only strong but if not corrected, could create tremendous problems in your mouth. If you are a chained smoker, the horrid smoke breath would definitely last over a period of time.

Many people who are dating have no idea that they have bad breath. Most people don't wake up in the morning and decide to test if they have bad breath. You would need someone among your circle of friends to tell you about it. Most of the time, it would require tremendous courage for your friends to tell you so.

If however, you date has bad breath, you should think about telling them. If you are really serious with the other person, you should try telling them honestly. This creates a space in your relationships where the other party knows that you are honest. They may even appreciate your honesty.

If you are someone with bad breath and your date feels the similar way, they may decide not to go out with you ever again.

You might be wondering why and having bad breath may be the reason. Ask someone close to you if it is so. If you really have bad breath, take the recommended actions.

Telling A Friend Or Family Member

Everyone on the planet have certain personal problems which they need to deal with. Some are more serious than others. Having bad breath is a serious condition and it would affect your social life tremendously.

Certain people may be affected seriously by your foul breath odour. Certain people just find it difficult to tell you what is wrong with you. They may feel that if they were to tell you about your bad breath problem, you may feel hurt by their honesty.

Different people deal with this condition differently. It is hard to say it in a manner which doesn't offend other people. Some people are very sensitive and would take heart to it.

However, there are methods in saying it in a contentious manner. You would need to do it in a manner which your relative or friend would understand what you are trying to say and that you don't hurt them.

However, you should be careful about your tone. Don't sound too abrasive or brash when talking to them. Among the main things that you should definitely not do include:

- Tell them directly that they have smell breath

- Ask them if they brush their teeth regularly
- Emphasize to them about their smelly breath
- Constantly repeat to them about their smelly breath
- Make offending gesture about their breath
- Make fun of them in front of other people

Be very considerate of their feelings. They may be going through some health issues and telling them directly that they have a smelly breath won't help at all. Everyone feels bad about their insecurities and adding this to that could only ignite more flames.

Talk to them normally. From there, you can ask if they have any oral health problems. Create an atmosphere where they are comfortable talking to you. They would give you either one of three responses: Yes, No or they might not want to talk about this.

If you get a yes, see if you can tell them more about this problem. If they say no, perhaps you can talk about the problem of halitosis. If their response is that they don't want to talk about it, perhaps you can wait for a time where you are comfortable talking about it.

If you have a chance to talk to them, let them know that this problem is related to their health. This isn't just a common health issue, but also a dental hygiene problem. Tell them that they can seek a doctor or dentist to help them with it.

Share with them the importance of brushing and flossing their teeth regularly. From here, they would know why it is so important.

Tell them that you are being frank because you want to help them. It may have impacted them socially in the past without them even knowing. Having bad breath is a big social problem. If you can get the message to them without them being offended, it is a great thing. Be there for them and don't hesitate to give more help if they need.

Resource 1 - Bad Breath Gone Quickly

Want to cure your bad breath in just 3 days?

You can read all about this special technique in The Bad Breath Report, a simple and straight-forward special report, in which you will also discover...

- **The single cause of virtually ALL cases of bad breath, and what you can do to control it, no matter how serious your problem, or how long you've had it.**

- 5 simple things you can do today that can rid you of bad breath, even before you try the treatment!

- **Brushing and flossing your teeth is good for you, but it will NOT improve your bad breath... find out why.**

- How to get rid of that ugly white coating on your tongue... without scraping!

This is a great report that you should definitely get. It has incredibly information that would shatter all the myths about curing bad breath permanently. Check it out:

http://badbreathgone.wellbeingvalley.com/

Resource 2 - The Myths Behind Bad Breath Cure

So, how would you like...

- **To never have to worry about your bad breath again, ever...**
- Breath which is not simply fresher, but likely to be even fresher than anybody else's that you will ever meet...
- **To improve your oral health so much your gums and teeth literally radiate health...**
- To stop wasting countless hours and dollars on ineffective cures...
- **To feel so happy and confident in yourself that you could literally**

grab and kiss the person you've been attracted to for the longest time...

- To begin to murder your bad breath and reclaim your life right now, literally...

And don't forget, the incredible part is all of this is down to a simple 3 minute routine in the morning. Check it out at:

http://badbreathcure.wellbeingvalley.com/